# The Fresh Factor

## A Proven System to Eliminating Body Odor and Living Confidently

### Christian Swan

# Copyright ©

Published by Christian Swan

© 2023

# Table Of Content

# Introduction

Have you ever found yourself feeling self-conscious about your body odor, wondering if everyone around you can smell it? Do you avoid social situations or physical activity because you're worried about how you'll smell? If so, you're not alone. Body odor is a common problem that affects millions of people worldwide.

However, the good news is that you don't have to live with body odor forever. With the right knowledge and tools, you can eliminate body odor and start living confidently. That's where this book comes in.

"The Fresh Factor: A Proven System to Eliminating Body Odor and Living Confidently" is your comprehensive guide to defeating body odor once and for all. Whether you're dealing with mild or severe body odor, this book has the solutions you need to stay fresh and confident in any situation.

In this book, we'll explore the science of body odor and what causes it, as well as the various types of body odor and what they mean. We'll also cover personal hygiene practices, dietary changes, natural remedies, sweat control methods, and more.

But this book isn't just about eliminating body odor. It's about empowering you to live confidently and without shame. We'll discuss the impact that body odor can have on your self-esteem and social life and provide strategies for overcoming the stigma and embracing your freshness.

Whether you're dealing with body odor yourself or trying to help someone else, "The Fresh Factor" is the ultimate guide to eliminating body odor and living confidently. With our proven system and expert advice, you can finally say goodbye to body odor and hello to a fresh, confident you.

# Chapter 1
## The Science of Body Odor: Understanding the Causes and Factors

Welcome to the first chapter of "The Fresh Factor: A Proven System to Eliminating Body Odor and Living Confidently". In this chapter, we'll dive deep into the science behind body odor and the factors that contribute to it. Let's get started!

So, what exactly is body odor? Simply put, it's the unpleasant smell that can come from your body. But what causes it? Well, the answer isn't quite as simple.

Body odor is primarily caused by the bacteria that live on our skin. These bacteria break down the sweat that our bodies produce, which can result in an unpleasant odor. But why do some people have more noticeable body odor than others?

Several factors can contribute to the severity of body odor. These include:

1.     Genetics: Believe it or not, some people are simply more prone to body odor than others due to their genetics. This is because certain genes can affect the type and amount of sweat that a person produces, which can in turn affect body odor.

2.     Diet: The food that we eat can also have an impact on our body odor. For example, eating spicy or strong-smelling foods can cause an odor to be more noticeable.

3.     Hormones: Hormonal changes in the body, such as those that occur during puberty or menopause, can also affect body odor.

4.     Medical Conditions: Certain medical conditions, such as diabetes, liver or kidney disease, and thyroid problems, can cause an increase in body odor.

Now that we've covered the factors that contribute to body odor, let's take a closer look at the types of body odor that can occur.

The most common types of body odor include.

1.    Axillary Odor: This is the type of body odor that occurs in the underarm area. This area is particularly prone to odor because it contains a high concentration of sweat glands.

2.    Foot Odor: Foot odor is caused by the same bacteria that cause axillary odor. When our feet sweat, the bacteria break down the sweat and create an unpleasant odor.

3.    Genital Odor: This type of body odor is caused by sweat and bacteria in the genital area.

So, now that we know what body odor is, what causes it, and the types that can occur, let's move on to the next question: How can we prevent it?

The good news is that there are many ways to prevent body odor. The most effective methods include:

1.      Good Personal Hygiene: This is perhaps the most important factor in preventing body odor. Regular showers, wearing clean clothes, and using deodorant or antiperspirant can all help to keep odor at bay.

2.      Dietary Changes: As we mentioned earlier, our diet can impact our body odor. Eating a healthy diet that's low in strong-smelling foods can help to reduce the severity of body odor.

3.      Natural Remedies: Many natural remedies can be used to fight body odor, such as baking soda, witch hazel, and apple cider vinegar.

4.      Sweat Control: Excessive sweating can contribute to body odor. Wearing breathable clothing, using sweat-wicking fabrics, and using antiperspirants can all help to control sweating and reduce odor.

In conclusion, body odor is a common problem that affects many people. However, with the right knowledge and tools, it's a problem that can be managed and even eliminated. By understanding the science behind body odor and the factors that contribute to it, we can take steps to prevent and control it. In the next chapter, we'll explore personal hygiene practices in more detail and provide tips for staying fresh and odor-free.

# Chapter 2

# Identifying Your Odor ~ Different Types of Body Odor and What They Mean

If you've ever struggled with body odor, you know that not all odors are created equal. Some smells are musty, while others are sour or even sweet. But did you know that the type of odor your body produces can reveal a lot about your health and lifestyle?

In this chapter, we'll explore the different types of body odor and what they mean. From musty to sour to sweet, we'll break down the science behind each smell and what it can reveal about your body.

## Musty Odor

A musty odor is one of the most common types of body odor. It's often described as a damp or stale smell, similar to that of a musty basement. This type of odor is caused by bacteria that thrive in warm, moist environments, such as the armpits or groin.

If you're experiencing a musty odor, it could be a sign that you're not drying off properly after showering or sweating. To combat this type of odor, make sure to towel dry thoroughly and apply a powder or antiperspirant to areas prone to moisture buildup.

## Sour Odor

A sour odor is another common type of body odor, and it's typically caused by the bacteria that thrive in sweat. This odor is often described as "sweaty" or "musky," and it can be quite pungent.

If you're experiencing a sour odor, it's important to remember that sweating is a natural bodily function. However, excessive sweating can exacerbate this type of odor. To combat sour body odor, try using a strong antiperspirant and wearing breathable clothing.

## Sweet Odor

While sweet body odor may sound pleasant, it's a sign of a potential health problem. This type of odor is often caused by a condition called diabetes mellitus, which affects how the body processes glucose.

If you're experiencing a sweet odor, it's important to speak with your doctor right away. Other symptoms of diabetes can include excessive thirst, frequent urination, and blurred vision.

## Fishy Odor

A fishy odor is a type of body odor that's often associated with vaginal health. It can be caused by a bacterial imbalance in the vagina, which can lead to an infection called bacterial vaginosis (BV).

If you're experiencing a fishy odor, it's important to see your gynecologist as soon as possible. BV is a common condition that affects many women, and it's easily treatable with antibiotics.

## Fecal Odor

While it may be unpleasant to talk about, fecal body odor is a real issue for some people. This type of odor is typically caused by poor hygiene practices, such as not wiping properly after using the bathroom.

If you're experiencing fecal body odor, it's important to improve your hygiene habits. Make sure to wipe thoroughly after using the bathroom and consider using wet wipes or a bidet to clean more effectively.

In conclusion, different types of body odor can reveal a lot about your health and lifestyle. If you're struggling with body odor, it's important to identify the type of odor you're experiencing and take steps to combat it. By using the right products, improving your hygiene practices, and speaking with your doctor, when necessary, you can eliminate body odor and live confidently.

# Chapter 3

## Personal Hygiene: Essential Practices to Keep Odor at Bay

Body odor is caused by the bacteria that live on our skin and feed on our sweat. When sweat accumulates on the skin, these bacteria break down the sweat and produce a foul-smelling odor. To keep body odor at bay, personal hygiene practices are essential.

In this chapter, we'll explore the importance of personal hygiene in preventing body odor and the specific practices you can incorporate into your daily routine to keep fresh and confident.

- **Daily Shower or Bath**

One of the most important hygiene practices to keep odor at bay is taking a shower or bath every day. This helps to remove sweat and bacteria from your skin's surface and keeps your body clean and fresh.

When taking a shower or bath, it's important to use a gentle soap that is free of harsh chemicals that can irritate the skin. Use warm water instead of hot water, as hot water can dry out the skin and cause irritation.

- **Properly Cleaning the Underarms**

The underarms are one of the most common areas where body odor occurs because they contain a high concentration of sweat glands. Therefore, it's essential to properly clean them to avoid the buildup of bacteria and sweat.

When washing your underarms, use a gentle soap and a washcloth or loofah to gently exfoliate the area. Be sure to rinse thoroughly to remove all soap residue.

- **Use of Antimicrobial Soap**

Antimicrobial soaps contain ingredients that kill bacteria, fungi, and viruses. They are effective in preventing the growth of bacteria on the skin and, therefore, reducing the risk of body odor.

However, it's important to note that overuse of antimicrobial soaps can lead to the development of resistant bacteria, which can be harmful to the body. Therefore, use antimicrobial soaps only as necessary, such as when traveling or in areas with poor hygiene.

- **Proper Use of Deodorants and Antiperspirants**

Deodorants and antiperspirants are essential tools in preventing body odor. Deodorants work by neutralizing the odor caused by bacteria on the skin, while antiperspirants work by reducing sweat production.

When using deodorants and antiperspirants, it's important to apply them correctly for maximum effectiveness. Apply deodorant to clean, dry underarms, and antiperspirant at night before bed to allow it to absorb fully into the skin.

- **Choosing the Right Clothing**

The clothes you wear can also affect body odor. Natural fibers, such as cotton and linen, are more breathable than synthetic fibers, which can trap sweat and bacteria.

In addition, wearing loose-fitting clothing allows air to circulate around your body and reduces sweat buildup. Avoid tight-fitting clothing, as it can trap sweat and bacteria and exacerbate body odor.

- **Practice Foot Hygiene**

Feet are another common area where body odor occurs due to the high concentration of sweat glands. To prevent foot odor, it's essential to practice good foot hygiene.

Wash your feet daily with soap and water and be sure to dry them thoroughly. Wear clean socks made of breathable material, such as cotton, and change them daily. Avoid wearing the same shoes every day, as this can cause a buildup of bacteria and sweat.

- **Hydrate Properly**

Drinking plenty of water is essential for overall health, but it also helps to prevent body odor. When you're dehydrated, your body produces less sweat, which can lead to a buildup of bacteria on the skin.

To avoid dehydration, drink at least eight glasses of water a day. You can also incorporate hydrating foods, such as watermelon, cucumber, and tomatoes, into your diet.

Personal hygiene plays a crucial role in keeping body odor at bay. It involves taking care of every part of your body regularly, from your hair down to your feet. It's not just about smelling good, but also about staying healthy and feeling confident.

Incorporating good personal hygiene practices into your daily routine may take some effort, but it's worth it. Not only will it help eliminate body odor, but it can also prevent other health problems like infections and skin irritations.

Remember, it's not just about using the right products and techniques, but also about being consistent with your hygiene habits. Make it a habit to clean yourself thoroughly every day, and don't forget to change your clothes and bedding regularly.

In the next chapter, we will discuss how your diet and nutrition choices can affect your body odor and what changes you can make to help control it.

# Chapter 4

# Diet and Nutrition: How Your Food Choices Affect Your Body Odor

What you eat can have a significant impact on your body odor. Certain foods and drinks can cause your body to produce strong and unpleasant odors, while others can help control it. In this chapter, we'll discuss the connection between your diet and body odor and provide you with tips on how to make healthier choices.

## The Science Behind It

Sweating is a natural process that helps regulate your body temperature. However, the sweat itself does not have an odor. The odor that we associate with sweat comes from the bacteria on our skin breaking down the sweat. This process creates a chemical reaction that produces a foul odor.

The foods we eat can affect the way our sweat smells. For example, foods high in sulfur, such as garlic and onions, can cause body odor to become more pungent. Similarly, foods high in protein, like red meat, can also make your sweat smell stronger.

On the other hand, some foods can help reduce body odor. Foods high in chlorophyll, such as leafy green vegetables like spinach and kale, can help neutralize body odor. Drinking plenty of water can also help flush toxins out of your body and reduce body odor.

**Tips for Making Healthier Food Choices**

1.     Avoid Foods High in Sulfur: As mentioned earlier, foods high in sulfur can cause body odor to become more pungent. Try to avoid or limit your intake of onions, garlic, and cruciferous vegetables like broccoli and cauliflower.

2.     Eat More Fresh Fruits and Vegetables: Fresh fruits and vegetables are packed with vitamins and minerals that can help keep your body healthy and reduce body odor. In particular, leafy greens like spinach, kale, and arugula contain chlorophyll, which can help neutralize body odor.

3.     Choose Lean Proteins: As much as possible, choose lean proteins like chicken, fish, and turkey. These meats are easier for your body to digest, and they don't produce as much sweat-inducing ammonia as red meat.

4.     Stay Hydrated: Drinking plenty of water can help flush toxins out of your body and reduce body odor. Aim for at least eight glasses of water a day and limit your intake of sugary drinks like soda and juice.

5.     Limit Alcohol and Caffeine: Alcohol and caffeine can cause your body to produce more sweat and make your sweat smell stronger. Limit your intake of these beverages and opt for water or herbal tea instead.

In addition to making healthier food choices, you can also supplement your diet with certain vitamins and minerals that can help control body odor. For example, taking a zinc supplement can help regulate your body's production of sweat and reduce body odor.

## Final Thoughts

In conclusion, what you eat can have a significant impact on your body odor. By making healthier food choices and supplementing your diet with the right vitamins and minerals, you can reduce body odor and feel more confident. Remember to stay hydrated, eat plenty of fresh fruits and vegetables, and limit your intake of foods high in sulfur, red meat, alcohol, and caffeine. With these tips, you can take control of your body odor and live more confidently.

# Chapter 5
## Natural Remedies ~ Home Remedies and Natural Products for Fighting Body Odor

Body odor can be a persistent and embarrassing problem for many individuals. Although deodorants and antiperspirants can help mask and control body odor, they often contain harsh chemicals that may cause irritation or have negative long-term effects on the body. For those who prefer a more natural approach to odor control, there are various home remedies and natural products that can be effective in fighting body odor.

- Apple cider vinegar: Apple cider vinegar has been used for centuries for various health benefits, including odor control. Its acidic properties make it an effective natural deodorant, as it can help eliminate odor-causing bacteria. Simply mix equal parts apple cider vinegar and water, apply the solution to a cotton pad, and wipe your underarms.

- Baking soda: Baking soda is another natural ingredient that can help neutralize odor. Its alkaline nature can help balance the pH level of the skin, making it less hospitable to odor-causing bacteria. Mix a tablespoon of baking soda with a little water to form a paste and apply it to your underarms. Leave it on for a few minutes before rinsing it off with water.

- Witch hazel: Witch hazel is a natural astringent that can help reduce sweat production, which in turn can help control body odor. Apply witch hazel to your underarms with a cotton ball, and let it dry before applying deodorant.

- Coconut oil: Coconut oil has natural antibacterial and antifungal properties that can help eliminate odor-causing bacteria. It can also help moisturize the skin and prevent irritation. Simply apply a small amount of coconut oil to your underarms and allow it to absorb before putting on clothes.

- Tea tree oil: Tea tree oil has antibacterial and antifungal properties that can help fight odor-causing bacteria. Mix a few drops of tea tree oil with carrier oil, such as coconut oil or olive oil, and apply the solution to your underarms.

- Lemon juice: Lemon juice has acidic properties that can help eliminate bacteria and reduce odor. Squeeze a lemon and apply the juice to your underarms using a cotton ball. Leave it on for a few minutes before rinsing it off with water.

- Sage: Sage is a herb that has natural antiperspirant properties and can help reduce sweat production. Brew a cup of sage tea and apply it to your underarms with a cotton ball. Allow it to dry before putting on clothes.

- Charcoal: Activated charcoal is a natural absorbent that can help eliminate odor-causing bacteria. It can be used in various forms, such as a powder or in a deodorant stick. Simply apply it to your underarms and let it absorb before putting on clothes.

- Cornstarch: Cornstarch is a natural absorbent that can help reduce moisture and odor. Apply it to your underarms with a powder puff or cotton ball.

- Essential oils: Essential oils such as lavender, peppermint, and eucalyptus have natural antibacterial properties and can help fight odor-causing bacteria. Mix a few drops of essential oil with carrier oil and apply the solution to your underarms.

It's important to note that natural remedies may not be as long-lasting or effective as commercial products and may require more frequent application throughout the day. Additionally, it's always best to test any new natural remedy on a small patch of skin before using it regularly.

In conclusion, natural remedies can be a great alternative to commercial products for individuals looking for a more natural approach to odor control.

With a little experimentation, you can find a natural remedy that works best for you and your body.

# Chapter 6

## Sweat Control: Managing Excessive Sweating and Its Impact on Body Odor

Sweating is a natural process that helps regulate body temperature and keep the body cool. However, excessive sweating can be a problem, especially when it leads to body odor. Excessive sweating is also known as hyperhidrosis, a condition that affects millions of people worldwide. In this chapter, we'll explore the causes of excessive sweating, its impact on body odor, and how to manage it.

**Causes of Excessive Sweating**

- Excessive sweating can be caused by various factors, including genetics, medical conditions, and medications. In some cases, there may not be an underlying cause. Here are some of the most common causes of excessive sweating:

- Genetics: Excessive sweating can run in families. If one or both of your parents have hyperhidrosis, you may also develop it.

- Medical conditions: Medical conditions such as thyroid problems, diabetes, and menopause can cause excessive sweating.

- Medications: Certain medications, such as antidepressants and blood pressure medications, can cause excessive sweating as a side effect.

- Anxiety and stress: Anxiety and stress can trigger excessive sweating in some people.

## Impact of Excessive Sweating on Body Odor

Excessive sweating can lead to an increase in body odor, especially in areas where sweat accumulates, such as the armpits and groin. Sweat itself is odorless, but when it comes into contact with bacteria on the skin's surface, it can produce an unpleasant smell. The bacteria break down the sweat, producing compounds that give off an odor.

## Managing Excessive Sweating

If you're experiencing excessive sweating, there are several ways to manage it. Here are some of the most effective methods:

- Antiperspirants: Antiperspirants are designed to reduce sweating by blocking the sweat glands' openings. They contain aluminum-based compounds that form a plug over the sweat gland openings, reducing the amount of sweat that is released. Antiperspirants are available in various forms, including roll-ons, sprays, and creams.

- Prescription antiperspirants: For more severe cases of hyperhidrosis, prescription-strength antiperspirants may be recommended. These antiperspirants contain higher concentrations of aluminum-based compounds and are more effective than over-the-counter products.

- Botox injections: Botox injections are a treatment option for excessive sweating. The injections work by blocking the nerve signals that stimulate the sweat glands, reducing sweating in the treated area.

- Medications: In some cases, medications may be prescribed to treat excessive sweating. These medications work by reducing the activity of the sweat glands.

- Iontophoresis: Iontophoresis is a non-invasive treatment that involves exposing the affected area to a low-level electrical current while immersed in water. The current blocks the sweat glands, reducing sweating.

- Surgery: In severe cases of hyperhidrosis, surgery may be recommended. The surgery involves removing the sweat glands in the affected area.

**Preventing Body Odor Caused by Excessive Sweating**

In addition to managing excessive sweating, there are steps you can take to prevent body odor caused by sweating. Here are some tips:

1.      Practice good personal hygiene: Shower or bathe at least once a day to remove bacteria and sweat from the skin's surface.

2.      Wear breathable clothing: Choose clothing made from natural fibers.

3.      Medications: In some cases, medications may be used to control excessive sweating. The most common medications used for this purpose are anticholinergics, which work by blocking the action of the neurotransmitter acetylcholine, which is responsible for activating sweat glands.

Anticholinergics can be taken orally or applied topically to the skin. However, they can cause side effects such as dry mouth, constipation, and blurred vision.

Other medications that may be used for sweat control include beta-blockers, which can reduce sweating by decreasing heart rate and blood pressure, and benzodiazepines, which can help reduce anxiety-related sweating.

4.     Surgery: In severe cases of excessive sweating, surgery may be necessary. One type of surgery commonly used for this purpose is called sympathectomy, which involves cutting or clamping the sympathetic nerves that control sweating in the affected area.

Sympathectomy is typically only used as a last resort when other treatments have failed, as it carries a risk of complications such as nerve damage and excessive sweating in other parts of the body.

Conclusion

Excessive sweating can be a frustrating and embarrassing problem, but it is also a treatable one. There are a variety of methods available for sweat control, ranging from simple lifestyle changes to more invasive medical procedures.

If you are struggling with excessive sweating, it is important to talk to your doctor about your options for sweat control. With the right treatment plan, you can regain your confidence and enjoy a more comfortable and sweat-free life.

# Chapter 7

## Deodorants and Antiperspirants: Understanding the Differences and Finding the Right Product for You

Deodorants and antiperspirants are popular personal care products used to combat body odor. While these two products are often used interchangeably, they are not the same thing. Understanding the differences between deodorants and antiperspirants is crucial in choosing the right product for your needs. In this chapter, we'll explore the differences between deodorants and antiperspirants, how they work, and what to look for when choosing the right product.

### Deodorants

Deodorants are products designed to mask and eliminate odor-causing bacteria on the skin. They contain antimicrobial agents that kill the bacteria responsible for body odor. Additionally, deodorants contain fragrances that help to cover up any residual odor.

Deodorants can come in many different forms, including sprays, roll-ons, sticks, and creams. Some deodorants also contain additional ingredients that offer other benefits, such as moisturizing agents for dry skin or skin conditioners to soothe irritation.

While deodorants are effective at masking and eliminating odor, they do not prevent sweating. For individuals who sweat heavily, a deodorant alone may not be enough to combat body odor. In this case, an antiperspirant may be necessary.

## Antiperspirants

Antiperspirants are products designed to prevent or reduce sweating. They contain aluminum-based compounds that work by forming a plug in the sweat glands, preventing sweat from reaching the skin's surface. By reducing the amount of sweat produced, antiperspirants also reduce the number of bacteria that can cause body odor.

Antiperspirants come in many different forms, including sprays, roll-ons, sticks, and creams. Some antiperspirants also contain additional ingredients that offer other benefits, such as moisturizing agents.

When selecting a deodorant or antiperspirant, it is important to consider the active ingredients, the scent, and any potential side effects. Some people may be sensitive to certain ingredients, such as aluminum or fragrances, and may need to opt for a natural or hypoallergenic option.

It is also important to keep in mind that deodorants and antiperspirants are not interchangeable. Deodorants are designed to mask odors and often contain antimicrobial agents to kill odor-causing bacteria. Antiperspirants, on the other hand, are designed to reduce sweat production by blocking the sweat ducts with aluminum-based compounds.

While antiperspirants may be effective in reducing sweating, some people may be concerned about the potential health risks associated with aluminum exposure. However, the American Cancer Society states that there is no conclusive evidence linking the use of antiperspirants or deodorants with an increased risk of breast cancer.

Overall, the choice between deodorant and antiperspirant is a personal one and may depend on individual preferences and needs. Some people may choose to use both for maximum odor and sweat protection.

When applying deodorant or antiperspirant, it is important to follow the instructions and apply it to clean dry skin. Applying it to wet or sweaty skin may decrease its effectiveness and cause skin irritation. It is also important to avoid overuse, as this can lead to clogged pores and skin irritation.

In addition to traditional deodorants and antiperspirants, there are also natural options available. These products often use plant-based ingredients such as tea tree oil, witch hazel, and baking soda to eliminate odors and control sweating.

It is important to note that natural deodorants may not be as effective as traditional options, particularly in situations of heavy sweating or intense physical activity. However, they can be a good option for those with sensitive skin or concerns about using products with synthetic ingredients.

In conclusion, deodorants and antiperspirants are important tools in controlling body odor and sweat. When selecting a product, it is important to consider individual needs and preferences, as well as potential side effects. With proper use and care, these products can help individuals feel fresh and confident throughout the day.

# Chapter 8

## Clothing and Laundry: Tips for Reducing Odor Buildup in Clothes

In addition to personal hygiene, the clothes you wear can also contribute to body odor. Sweat and bacteria can build up on your clothes, leading to unpleasant odors. Here are some tips for reducing odor buildup in your clothes:

1.     Choose the Right Fabrics: Some fabrics are more breathable than others, which can help reduce odor buildup. Natural fibers like cotton, linen, and wool are more breathable than synthetic materials like polyester and nylon. Choose clothes made from natural fibers when possible, especially for items like underwear and socks.

2.     Wash Clothes Regularly: Washing your clothes regularly is essential for preventing odor buildup. Sweaty clothes should be washed as soon as possible to prevent bacteria from multiplying. It's also important to wash clothes after each wear, especially if you've been sweating or exercising.

3.	Use the Right Laundry Detergent: Using a laundry detergent that's designed to remove odors can help keep your clothes smelling fresh. Look for detergents that are specifically formulated for sports or workout clothes, as they're designed to remove sweat and odor buildup.

4.	Don't Overload the Washing Machine: Overloading the washing machine can prevent clothes from getting clean and can contribute to odor buildup. Follow the manufacturer's instructions for the maximum load size and don't exceed it.

5.	Use Hot Water: Hot water can help kill bacteria and remove odor buildup. Use the hottest water recommended for your clothing and consider using a sanitizing cycle if your washing machine has one.

6.	Don't Leave Wet Clothes in the Washer: Leaving wet clothes in the washing machine can lead to mildew and odor buildup. Be sure to remove clothes promptly and dry them as soon as possible.

7.      Dry Clothes Thoroughly: Drying clothes thoroughly is important for preventing odor buildup. Make sure clothes are completely dry before storing them, as damp clothes can lead to mildew and musty odors. Consider using a dryer sheet or fabric softener to help clothes smell fresh.

8.      Air Out Clothes: If possible, hang clothes outside to air out before storing them. Fresh air can help remove odors and keep clothes smelling fresh.

9.      Store Clothes Properly: Proper storage can help prevent odor buildup in clothes. Make sure clothes are completely dry before storing them, and store them in a cool, dry place. Avoid storing clothes in damp or humid areas, as this can lead to mildew and musty odors.

By following these tips, you can help reduce odor buildup in your clothes and keep them smelling fresh. Remember, personal hygiene and clothing care go hand in hand when it comes to preventing body odor.

# Chapter 9

# Managing Odor in Specific Situations: Odor Management for Exercise, Stress, and Other Factors

Body odor can be a challenge to manage, especially in specific situations that can trigger excessive sweating and odor production. These situations may include exercise, stress, and other factors that can cause us to sweat more than usual. In this chapter, we will discuss ways to manage odor in these specific situations.

## Exercise and Body Odor

Exercise is great for our physical and mental health, but it can also be a trigger for body odor. When we exercise, our body temperature rises, causing us to sweat more. This sweats mixes with the bacteria on our skin, creating a strong odor.

To manage body odor during exercise, there are a few things you can do. First, make sure to wear breathable, moisture-wicking clothing that can help absorb sweat and prevent it from lingering on your skin. Second, shower immediately after your workout to remove any sweat and bacteria that may have built up. Third, use antiperspirant before your workout to help reduce sweating and odor.

If you're exercising outdoors in hot weather, it's especially important to stay hydrated. Drinking plenty of water can help regulate your body temperature and reduce excessive sweating.

## Stress and Body Odor

Stress is another factor that can trigger body odor. When we're stressed, our bodies produce more sweat, which can lead to an increase in odor-causing bacteria.

To manage body odor during times of stress, there are a few things you can do. First, try to manage your stress levels by practicing relaxation techniques, such as meditation or yoga. When you're relaxed, your body produces less sweat and therefore less odor.

Second, make sure to wear breathable clothing that can help absorb sweat and prevent it from lingering on your skin. Third, shower regularly and use an antiperspirant to help reduce sweating and odor.

## Other Factors and Body Odor

Other factors can trigger body odor, such as certain medications and medical conditions. If you're taking medication that is causing you to sweat more than usual or produce a strong odor, talk to your doctor about possible alternatives.

Certain medical conditions, such as hyperhidrosis (excessive sweating) or trimethylaminuria (a metabolic disorder that causes a fishy odor), can also cause body odor. If you're experiencing persistent body odor despite your best efforts to manage it, talk to your doctor to rule out any underlying medical conditions.

## Final Thoughts

Managing body odor can be challenging, but with the right strategies and tools, it's possible to stay fresh and confident in any situation. Whether you're dealing with excessive sweating, stress, or other factors that can trigger body odor, there are steps you can take to manage it.

Remember to practice good personal hygiene, eat a healthy diet, use natural remedies, and choose the right products, such as antiperspirants and deodorants, to help control body odor. And don't be afraid to talk to your doctor if you're experiencing persistent body odor that is impacting your daily life. With the right support and guidance, you can overcome body odor and live confidently.

# Chapter 10
## Odor and Self~Confidence: Overcoming the Stigma and Embracing Your Freshness

Body odor can be embarrassing and can negatively affect one's self-confidence. It's not uncommon for individuals to feel self-conscious and ashamed about their body odor, which can lead to avoiding social situations, intimacy, and physical activities. However, it's important to remember that body odor is a natural occurrence and is experienced by many individuals. In this chapter, we will discuss the impact of body odor on self-confidence and strategies for overcoming the stigma and embracing your freshness.

### The Impact of Body Odor on Self-Confidence

Body odor can significantly impact an individual's self-confidence. It can cause them to feel embarrassed and ashamed, leading to low self-esteem and a lack of confidence in their abilities. This can be particularly challenging in situations where body odor is more noticeable, such as in public places, at work, or during physical activities.

Individuals with body odor may find themselves avoiding social situations, relationships, and physical activities due to their fear of being judged or ridiculed. This can have a negative impact on their mental health and overall well-being, leading to feelings of isolation, anxiety, and depression.

## Overcoming the Stigma and Embracing Your Freshness

Overcoming the stigma associated with body odor can be challenging, but it's important to remember that it's a natural occurrence and that there are ways to manage it. Here are some strategies to help you overcome the stigma and embrace your freshness:

1. Develop a Positive Mindset: It's important to develop a positive mindset and remind yourself that body odor is natural and can be managed. Focus on your strengths and abilities rather than your perceived flaws.

2.    Practice Good Hygiene: Maintaining good personal hygiene is essential for managing body odor. Bathe regularly, use mild soap, and wear clean clothes. Don't forget to apply deodorant or antiperspirant.

3.    Choose the Right Clothing: Certain fabrics can trap odors, so it's important to choose clothes made from breathable materials such as cotton, linen, or rayon. Avoid tight-fitting clothes, as they can cause sweating and make body odor worse.

4.    Be Mindful of Your Diet: What you eat can affect your body odor. Avoid foods with strong odors, such as garlic and onions, and drink plenty of water to help flush out toxins.

5.    Use Natural Remedies: Natural remedies such as tea tree oil and witch hazel can be effective in managing body odor. These products have antimicrobial properties that help kill bacteria that cause odor.

6.    Seek Professional Help: If you have tried these strategies and are still experiencing body odor, it may be time to seek professional help. A

dermatologist can prescribe medications or recommend treatments such as Botox injections to manage excessive sweating.

7.      Be Confident: The key to overcoming the stigma associated with body odor is to be confident in yourself. Remember that everyone has flaws, and it's important to embrace your uniqueness. Be proud of who you are and don't let body odor define you.

Body odor can be embarrassing and negatively impact an individual's self-confidence. However, it's important to remember that it's a natural occurrence and can be managed. By developing a positive mindset, practicing good hygiene, choosing the right clothing, being mindful of your diet, using natural remedies, seeking professional help when needed, and being confident in yourself, you can overcome the stigma associated with body odor and embrace your freshness. Remember, everyone has flaws, and it's important to embrace your uniqueness and be proud of who you are.

www.ingramcontent.com/pod-product-compliance
Lightning Source LLC
Chambersburg PA
CBHW061556250726
48657CB00021B/2054